CW01081644

All Ab
MANAGING VENOUS ULCERS

By V. M. Taylor in consultation with Alan Neil, Lisa Ovington, PhD, and Dr. Louis Grondin.

Our thanks also to the WOCN (Wound Ostomy Continence Nurses) members and members of CAET (Canadian Association of Enterostomal Nurses) who assisted in the editing and feedback survey pertaining to this book.

ISBN # 978 1 896616 85 8

Venous ulcers. Venous Leg Ulcers. Preventing venous ulcers. Leg ulcers care. Skin care for ulcers.

The publisher, Mediscript Communications Inc., acknowledges the financial support of the Government of Canada through the Book Publishing Industry Development Program (BPIDP) for our publishing activities.

Printed in Canada

www.mediscript.net

Book and Front Cover design by:
Brian Adamson, www.AdamsonGraphics.net

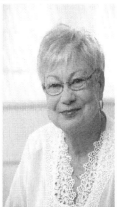

CONTENTS

INTRODUCTION

This book provides basic, non controversial and trusted information that can help a wide spectrum of readers.

The primary objective of the information is to help a person provide effective quality care to a loved one or someone in his or her care.

Your role as a caregiver could mean the older person in your care is a family member or loved one, or you may be a non family member who is helping out a friend. Alternatively, you may be a paid health worker providing quality care for a client. With this in mind, we will alternate between referring to family members, loved ones, older persons and clients.

All the information is reliable and was written by a group of eminent nurse educators who ensured the information complies with best practice guidelines and satisfies the various accreditation and regulatory bodies. Because there is so much unreliable information on the internet, you can be assured the "All About" publications are HON (Health On the Net) certified.

AN IMPORTANT MESSAGE FROM THE PUBLISHER

Each person's treatment, advice, medical aids, physical therapy and other approaches to health care are unique and highly dependant upon the diagnosis and overall assessment by the medical team.

We emphasize therefore that the information within this book is not a substitute for the advice and treatment from a health care professional.

This book provides generic information concerning venous ulcers, the causes and symptoms, and common sense well established care practices for caring for people with the condition.

With all this in mind, the publishers and authors disclaim any responsibility for any adverse effects resulting directly or indirectly from the suggestions contained within this book or from any misunderstanding of the content on the part of the reader.

HAVE YOU HEARD

The following notices were found in various locations:

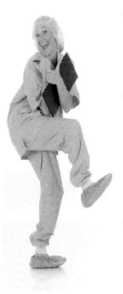

- Sign in a maternity clothing store: "We are open on labor day."

- In the vestry of a New England church: "Will the last person to leave please see that the perpetual light is extinguished?"

- In the window of an Oregon store: "Why go elsewhere and be cheated when you can come here?"

HOW MUCH DO YOU KNOW?

It helps to figure out how much you know before you start. In this way you will have an idea as to the gaps in your knowledge prior to reading the content. Please circle to indicate the best answer. Remember, at this stage, you are not expected to know all the answers:

1. What does the word venous specifically refer to?

a. Blood circulation

b. Skin breakdown

c. Pertaining to the veins

d. Stockings or bandages

2. Which of the following ulcers is NOT classified as an exclusive leg ulcer?

a. Arterial

b. Pressure

c. Venous

d. Diabetic

3. Which is the most common type of chronic skin ulcer?

a. Arterial

b. Diabetic

c. Venous

d. Pressure

4. Which of the following is NOT a quality of life issue for a venous ulcer sufferer?

a. Pain and discomfort

b. Embarrassment over a possible bad odor

c. Confidence to socialize with other clients

d. Inability to exercise properly

5. Where is the most common site for a venous leg ulcer to develop?

a. On the inside of the leg above the ankle

b. Both the foot and ankle

c. Close to a visible vein

d. Anywhere on the leg

6. Which of the following does NOT provide symptomatic relief from a venous ulcer?

a. Elevating the leg

b. Standing still to ease blood flow

c. Compression bandages

d. Compression stockings

7. What is NOT the function of compression hosiery/ stockings?

a. Provide pressure around the legs

b. Reduce swelling around the legs

c. Assist the venous blood flow back to the heart

d. Provide some aesthetic help with varicose veins

ANSWERS

1. c. The word venous pertains to the veins.

2. b. Pressure ulcers are caused by pressure points mostly on bony prominences of the skin and can occur on many different parts of the body.

3. c. Venous leg ulcers are the most common type of chronic leg ulcers – approximately 70% of leg ulcers are the venous type.

4. d. While exercise helps to improve blood circulation and contributes to a feeling of well-being, the pain of an ulcer, embarrassment over possible odor, and lack of confidence when it comes to socializing have much greater impact on a person's quality of life.

5. a. Venous leg ulcers commonly develop on the inside of the leg above the ankle.

6. b. Standing still to ease blood flow actually causes the blood to "pool" into the lower leg, contributing to the problem.

7. d. Compression hosiery/stockings are not specifically designed to provide aesthetic help with varicose veins. Although the person wearing them may perceive this as true, it is not an actual therapeutic function.

ABOUT VENOUS ULCERS

There are three types of leg ulcers: diabetic, arterial and venous.

It is estimated that about 70-90% of all leg ulcers are of the venous type cause by blood circulation problems. Venous leg ulcers are therefore the most common and studies have estimated that venous ulcers occur in 1-2% of the population – in other words, about 500,000 North Americans suffer from venous ulcers. Approximately 2/3 of people who develop a venous leg ulcer will go on to develop at least one more.

A venous ulcer can be a serious problem, best described as an open wound which can affect the deeper skin layers.

Venous leg ulcer sufferers can have their quality of life significantly affected; venous ulcers cause discomfort, pain and emotional distress, they lead to absence of work and can become a social disability due to embarrassing odors associated with the ulcers.

The good news is that, of all the different types of leg ulcers, the venous type is the most receptive to better lifestyle and self care practices so it is vital that the patient and caregiver strive to comply with both treatment and self help issues.

A venous ulcer can become a chronic problem where complete healing is difficult to achieve. This provides extra incentive to prevent venous ulcers from occurring in the first place, if possible.

New treatments, maintaining good self care habits and overall support for sufferers are helping to turn things around.

The purpose of this book is to help you understand how a venous ulcer develops, taking into account the various risk factors so that you can take actions to prevent one forming. If you are caring for someone with a venous ulcer, the various treatments and self care practices are highlighted to ensure healing takes place as quickly as possible.

SOMETHING TO THINK ABOUT...

The size of your body is of
little account;
the size of your brain
is of much account;
the size of your heart is of
the most account of all.

B. C. Forbes

CAUSES OF VENOUS LEG ULCERS

By understanding what causes venous leg ulcers can help in both preventing them and helping them to heal.

BLOOD FLOW IN THE LEG

The basic reason for venous ulcers developing is the lack of oxygen and nutrients reaching a damaged area of the skin on the leg, delaying the healing process. Blood flow carrying oxygen and nutrients in the leg is the critical factor so it is important to understand the blood flow (circulatory system) with the legs.

Two types of vessels carry blood throughout the body:

Arteries

Arteries carry blood rich in oxygen from the heart to all parts of the body including the legs. These arteries have muscular walls which can squeeze the blood onwards through its own contractions. These arteries break down into smaller (narrower) components often called arterioles or capillaries to ensure the extremities of the body receive oxygen and nutrients, which in turn provide all the energy and material necessary for the cells to stay healthy.

Veins

Veins carry the blood that has given up its oxygen and nutrients to the cells of the body and return this depleted blood back to the heart and then on to the lungs for replenishment of oxygen and so the cycle continues. Unlike the arteries, the veins do not have muscles to pump the blood forward. The veins have to rely on other methods to pump the blood such as muscles regularly squeezing the veins.

VEIN PROBLEMS CAUSE VENOUS ULCERS

The force generated by the heart cannot unassisted overcome the forces of gravity and drive the blood back from the legs to the heart. Consequently, another mechanism is involved where the calf muscles of the legs, when they contract, squeeze the deep veins of the leg and drive the blood forward.

Downward flow of the blood is prevented by the presence of valves found at regular intervals of the deep veins. These valves divide the veins into sections, each valve forming a "floor" to support the blood above it.

At the end of each heartbeat, the valves in the deep veins close to stop the blood flowing backward.

These deep veins are connected to one another by perforating veins which carry blood from a superficial vein (nearer the surface and thinner). When the perforating vein meets a deep vein, reverse flow is prevented by a one-way valve.

If and when the perforating vein valves fail, blood from the deep veins system is forced at high pressure into the superficial veins (near the skin surface). This causes the superficial veins to become congested and dilate, leading to the appearance of varicose veins, close to the surface of the skin.

Varicose veins are a very common condition and often minimal treatment is necessary but this is the first part of the process for people who eventually develop venous ulcers.

CHRONIC VENOUS INSUFFICIENCY (CVI)

This is the next step in the venous disease process that can lead to venous leg ulcers.

The continuing demise of the vein valves means that "high pressure" blood during the contraction phase of the calf muscle pumping blood from the deep veins to the superficial veins creates pressure that the smaller superficial veins cannot tolerate.

Extensive damage can be done to the delicate tissues including capillaries (tiny blood vessels).

In the end, the smooth transition of fluid and oxygen exchanges between the small blood vessels is impaired.

The most significant and visual aspect of this process is the blood "pooling" in the lower leg venous system causing swelling. The swelling (edema) of the tissues can cause more fluid and substances to accumulate resulting in less oxygen to the tissues. This lack of oxygen is the major contributor to the formation of a venous leg ulcer.

SYMPTOMS & CAUSE OF SYMPTOMS

SYMPTOM	CAUSE
Swelling (edema) in the legs and ankles	High venous pressure stretches vessels walls letting fluid leak out
Staining	High venous pressure stretches walls letting the red blood cells leak out
Pain when leg is down	Gravity pulls more blood down the leg
Pain relieved when leg is up	Gravity helps blood flow to the heart
Skin surface moist	Plenty of fluid in the area
Red surface	Lots of blood in the area, not moving properly
Tired, aching feeling	Too much blood in the vein causing increased pressure on the vein walls
Varicose vein appearance	Increase blood pressure in the vein causes stretching and twisting of the vein near the skin surface
Wound drainage	Leaking fluid in the area

A WORD ABOUT VARICOSE VEINS

Varicose veins are a very common condition, affecting 50% of the population in developed countries to some degree. The good news is that for at least 2/3 of the diagnosed varicose vein population, the condition is medically insignificant, meaning these people can live with the problem with no adverse health effects.

For the remaining third, varicose veins present a significant medical problem, giving rise to physical symptoms of heaviness and aching limbs, sometimes accompanied by cramps and swollen ankles.

Varicose veins can be a progressive condition. Once a vein has started to dilate, its walls become weak and its valves become dysfunctional, making the situation worse.

Treatment can be as simple as removing tight shoes, elevating the feet periodically, walking about frequently instead of constantly standing and wearing compression stockings. More serious cases could involve medical or surgical treatment.

Varicose veins are noticeable on the inner side of the leg, knee and thigh.

APPEARANCE

The symptoms of CVI can be subtle but there is no mistaking the arrival of the venous leg ulcer, which is often accompanied by a strong, offensive odor.

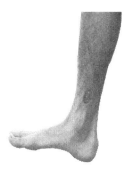

Usually it occurs on the inside surface of the leg just above the ankle. The shape is usually irregular and it can have a red or yellow coloring.

There is usually swelling (edema) around the lower leg area with some red or brownish staining.

One key indication that you have a venous leg ulcer is the relief of pain when the leg is elevated, i.e. when you are lying down and your legs are stretched out 6 inches above your heart.

DIAGNOSIS AND MONITORING

Observation alone permits diagnosis of an existing leg ulcer. Also, the symptoms listed previously can provide those all-important warnings that the person is at risk.

The physician and nurse have a range of objective ways of providing more in-depth information as to the nature of the problem; a commonly used test is the Doppler test to measure blood flow around the ankle, using a Doppler ultrasound device.

This device is the size of a large pen or pencil. It is used to listen to blood flow across your skin through the aid of a gel-like substance which is applied between the skin and the Doppler probe, which is a sort of sophisticated microphone.

The Doppler device is used for one of the most important blood circulatory diagnostic tests called the ANKLE BRACHIAL PRESSURE INDEX (ABPI) which tells the medical team how well your arteries are functioning. This is important because it allows the physician to determine how well fresh arterial (oxygenated) blood is getting to your legs and feet. With this information the medical team can decide on the appropriate treatment to heal the ulcer. More specifically, the physician can determine whether or not compression therapy should be used.

Aside from the Doppler and other tests, the medical team will keep records to monitor progress of the leg ulcer. By doing this, the progress of the ulcer can be evaluated and appropriate changes in treatment made to speed up healing.

This has to be done as objectively as possible, using measuring devices. A simple way is to use a ruler to measure the maximum and minimum widths. Alternatively, the outline of the ulcer can be traced on transparent material.

Here are some of the guidelines the medical team uses to document and subsequently monitor the ulcer:

Location	Edge characteristics
The history/duration	Size (depth, length and breadth)
Condition of surrounding skin	Amount of staining visible
Appearance of wound bed	Swelling
Nature of wound drainage	Amount/type of odour
Amount of pain/discomfort	Previous ulceration

RISK FACTORS

We now understand the way leg ulcers develop from varicose veins and chronic venous insufficiency—the breakdown of valves in the veins and the swelling of tissues and so on.

However, why this happens with certain individuals and not with others is more difficult to pinpoint.

A brief overview of risk factors is listed below; some of these you can do nothing about, while others can be controlled. Over the years, some of these risk factors may have contributed towards gradually developing CVI and the subsequent venous ulcer.

Occupations

Clients who had jobs which required long periods of standing, without muscular exertion: for example, hairdressers, pharmacists, factory workers, teachers, nurses, store clerks, and flight attendants.

Restrictive clothing

Tight clothing can have an adverse effect on blood circulation.

Pregnancy

Although the formation of varicose veins associated with pregnancy may be temporary, it has been shown the risk of developing varicose veins doubles with two or more pregnancies. In fact, it's estimated that up to 40% of all pregnant women develop varicose veins.

Trauma or injury

A knock or injury to the leg or ankle can damage the skin and contribute to an ulcer developing if someone is vulnerable to venous leg ulcer formation.

Overweight

Some studies suggest a link between being overweight (more specifically, being obese) and developing varicose veins. More weight puts above average pressure on the ankle joints, makes the heart work faster and contributes to high blood pressure. Also, being overweight means you have more blood and therefore the blood may "pool" in the lower legs.

Sedentary lifestyle

Reduced physical activity has long been associated with venous disease. Remember, the calf muscle is responsible for the pumping function that pushes up venous blood from the legs to the heart. Obviously, if these muscles are not used, the venous blood is going to collect or pool in the legs and venous pressure will increase in the legs. The message here is use those calf muscles. If you do not walk much, just moving your feet upwards can help.

Smoking cigarettes

As with so many illnesses, smoking cigarettes can worsen the condition. The role smoking plays in venous leg ulcers and venous disease is that of damaging the blood circulatory system. Smoking narrows arteries and reduces oxygen within the blood vessels making the skin unhealthy. If someone has a venous ulcer it slows down the healing process because less oxygen and healing nutrients are getting to the damaged skin.

Direct heat to the leg

Avoid strong, direct heat from a lamp or electric heater, jaccuzzi or very hot baths. Although it may feel good in the short term, this type of heat can further damage the skin or aggravate an existing leg ulcer.

Skin care

The skin is the part of the body that breaks down in a venous leg ulcer so it makes sense to try to keep it as healthy as possible so that it can defend itself against the venous blood circulation problems. The main objectives of skin care are to maintain soft, supple, clean and healthy skin and prevent irritation.

Heredity

One study found that the risk of developing venous disease was doubled for people with a relative with the condition.

Deep vein thrombosis (DVT)

This is a medical condition that can contribute to varicose veins and venous leg ulceration but it is difficult to diagnose and its true prevalence is difficult to estimate.

Aging

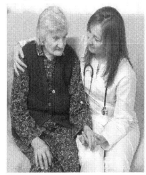

As venous disease is a progressive, time-driven, destructive process, it is natural that varicose veins and associated venous disease will get worse over time.

Adherence to treatment (compliance) and self care

Treatment – like compression bandaging and stockings as well as many self help tips like rest and elevation of the legs – requires the cooperation and motivation of the person if it is going to be truly effective.

RISK CHECKLIST

Risk Factor	Action Required
Restrictive clothing	
Avoiding standing for a long time	
Preventing injury or trauma	
Sedentary (not exercising)	
Direct heat to the leg	
Smoking cigarettes	
Preventative skin care	
Avoiding scratching	
Good hygiene	
Treatment compliance	

TREATMENT OPTIONS

Treatment of venous ulcers focuses on four separate but interrelated categories:

1. Compression to treat the Chronic Venous Insufficiency;
2. Wound care - the ulcer surface;
3. Surrounding skin care, and
4. Treatment of pain associated with the ulcer.

1. COMPRESSION

Swelling (edema) is primarily caused by high venous pressure. High blood pressure in the veins is also known as venous hypertension.

Compression bandaging

It is widely recognized and documented that venous leg ulcers require compression of the lower leg to heal effectively. Compression reduces the swelling (edema) in the lower leg, reduces pain, and helps the blood to move out of the leg back to the heart.

Compression provides a counter force to venous hypertension and forces small blood vessels to shrink back to normal so that fluid and cells no longer leak out of the blood vessels and oxygen and nutrients can be transported in the normal fashion.

Compression is required to aid the restoration of normal blood flow to the lower leg. Before healing can occur, it is necessary to reduce the swelling (edema) in the leg.

There are two types of compression used: rigid bandages (short stretch) have little stretching capacity, while elastic bandages (long stretch) are less rigid and contain more stretching capacity.

Rigid (inelastic) compression

Unna's Boot

In this common form of treatment, a moist bandage is wrapped around the lower leg and covered with another bandage to keep the moist bandage protected from soiling. The moist bandage usually contains a zinc oxide base and may contain other ingredients to assist in providing moisture and reduce skin irritation.

It is important to remember that the Unna's Boot works best when combined with exercise such as walking. One should stay active and not expect the bandage to do all the work.

There are other types of rigid compression treatments but this is the most common.

Elastic compression

You can recognize elastic bandages by the way they stretch and pull back when you release them. Elastic bandages supply pressure to the leg when applied. They work with your muscle pumps and provide constant compression when exercising. They are designed to provide an external counter pressure that works to reduce the effect of the high venous pressure that led to the ulcer.

There are two main types of elastic bandages to treat venous ulcers: moderate compression elastic and high compression elastic.

Elastic bandages may also be used in the new multi-layered compression systems.

High compression elastic bandages feel strong when you stretch them and may have little squares or indicators that allow you to determine when you have stretched them properly.

They are often applied by themselves over a padding bandage. They may need to be removed at night and put on again first thing in the morning. Some bandaging systems may be worn for up to a full week. A health care professional will be the one to determine how long to wear the compression bandaging system.

Moderate compression bandages do not feel as strong when you pull them on and usually don't supply enough compression when used alone. They are often used as part of a multi-layer compression system which allows continued compression even after the swelling subsides.

Several multi-layer compression systems are available that take advantage of the different properties of individual layers. They may vary in layers; some contain three while others contain four. Most are left on for up to a week to keep the leg under continuous compression.

One might think that because of all the pressure they put on the leg, compression bandages would be uncomfortable. In fact, most people find they are more comfortable and have less pain when their leg is under compression. By providing a counter pressure to the venous hypertension, they keep swelling down, improve the blood flow to the leg and reduce the damage and pain caused by the stretching of the blood vessels.

Key principles of compression bandaging:

- Compression bandaging should not be used if there is arterial disease and leg ulcers. More damage can occur in the ulcer or within the blood circulation system.

- There should be graduated compression – greatest at the ankle while decreasing as it is applied up the leg. Compression is measured in millimeters (mm) of mercury (Hg). Although everyone's needs are different, the general rule is 32 to 42 mm Hg at the ankle (if tolerated) and ending with 12 to 17 mmHg below the knee.

- Overly tight bandaging should be avoided. This may cause too much constriction resulting in persistent pain.

- Compression to the ulcerated area alone is ineffective.

- The bandage must be applied from the toe to the knee, molding around the ankle, up to the level just below the knee.

- The bandage must not be applied directly to the ulcer or to skin which is damaged or inflamed. A dressing or a paste bandage must act as a buffer.

- After healing, further compression may be necessary to prevent recurrence. At this point a compression stocking may be appropriate.

- Co-operation on the part of the patient is absolutely vital when using a compression bandage. For example, the elevation of the legs just above the heart helps the compression treatment.

Compression hosiery (stockings)

Compression hosiery works collaboratively with the calf muscles for a dual effect, which helps the venous valves to close. The weave and the fabric of each stocking create slight recoil tension, thereby exerting a constant, gently pressure on the limb.

The action of the stocking pushes inwards onto the limb, while the calf muscles push outwards. The benefit of this dual effect assists the venous valves to close and sufficiently return blood and fluids back to the heart.

Additionally, the stocking prevents further fluid build up. Pain and swelling are reduced and comfort is improved, while further ulcer development is avoided.

There is a wide range of compression hosiery available in different brands, shapes, sizes and styles. Compression hosiery comes in knee-high, thigh-high, and full pantyhose styles. It is important to choose the appropriate compression in order to achieve consistent therapeutic benefit.

Four Categories of Compression Hosiery

1) Support Wear:

Contains a very mild compression of 8-5 mmHg

• Tired aching legs

• Mild swelling

• Prevention for people who are required to stand or sit in one position for long periods of time.

2) Medical Leg Wear:

Available in compressions from 15-50 mmHg

• Management and prevention of venous leg ulcer minor to severe varicosities

• Minor to severe edema (swelling)

• Post-surgery and sclerotherapy (veins removed)

• Pregnancy related edema and varicosities

• Lymphatic edema

• Management of Chronic Venous Insufficiency

3) Custom Wear:

Available in compression of 15-90 mmHg

• Patients with abnormal limb shapes

• Patients who need an unlimited size range

• Patients who need specific garment options to improve compliance and fit

- Patients who need long-term management of lyphedema or vascular edema

4) **Ulcer Care:**

Contains a compression of 40 mmHg

- Designed specifically for use with venous ulcerations

- Two-part system providing a total pressure of 40+ mmHg

- Liner holds dressing in place, is easy to put one, is worn 24 hours a day, facilitates donning of outer stocking

- Is used until the ulceration heals

- Outer stocking has zipper to facilitate donning and is worn during ambulation over the white liner

- Open toe stocking

The venous hypertension which caused the leg ulcer does not go away. Once the ulcer has healed, the person will need to wear these stockings as a preventive measure in order to keep compression on the leg whenever they are not lying down.

As with a compression bandage, the correct fitting of the stocking by a professional is vital for a successful health outcome.

A follow-up appointment is usually arranged after the

hosiery has been fitted to ensure that the stocking is being used properly. Regular review may be required to check for any problems.

Ideally, new hosiery should be re-ordered every four to six months.

DID YOU KNOW

- Compression stockings DO NOT damage blood circulation; on the contrary they assist venous circulation in the legs.

- Compression stockings DO NOT weaken the muscles in the leg. Walking will provide the exercise to maintain muscle tone.

- The main purpose of compression hosiery is to prevent leg ulcers and avoid recurrence. It is also used to reduce venous hypertension on a sustained long term basis.

Here are the instructions for wearing stockings:

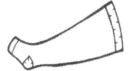

1. Your stocking.

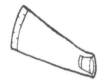

2. turn stocking inside out up to heel.

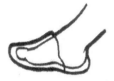

3. Place your slipper over your foot.

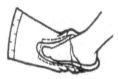

4. Pull foot of stocking over your foot.

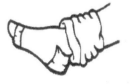

5. Slowly ease stocking up over heel and ankle.

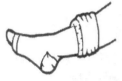

6. Gently ease the rest of the stocking a bit at a time up the leg

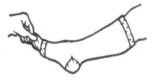

7. Pull slipper liner through the opening of the toes.

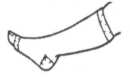

8. if this is a knee length stocking, the top should go no further than the crease behind your knee.

There should be no creases or wrinkles. The stocking should fit smoothly along the leg.

2. WOUND CARE: The ulcer surface

Though maintaining proper compression is the key to healing your venous leg ulcer you will also need to take care of the actual wound as it heals. Nature sets a healing time for each type of wound but that healing will only occur if there are favorable conditions for the ulcer to heal. Wounds must be kept clean (free from debris and infection), warm (not hot), protected from the outside environment and allowed to stay moist (not wet).

For your information these are the steps that can be taken in ulcer care:

Cleansing

Most of the time the medical team will rinse the ulcer surface with a simple salt (saline) solution. This will be formulated to be as close as possible to the normal salt concentration in your body fluids.

Debridement

This is the term used for the physical removal of any blood clots, scabs or dry crust on the ulcer through mechanical, chemical or surgical means.

Antibiotics or antimicrobials

These may be used to clear up an infection within the ulcer. A topical antibiotic may be applied to the ulcer surface and or it may be taken orally.

Drug therapy

Other than antibiotics there are few drugs that can improve the healing. Pain killers (analgesics) may be prescribed or recommended.

3. SKIN CARE

The goals of good skin care, especially for the area around the ulcer, are:

• Maintain soft, supple, clean and healthy skin.

• Prevent skin irritation and subsequent damage.

The use of proper skin care products provides enormous preventative and healing benefits for the patient with fragile and compromised skin.

Some of these products may include:

• A cleanser that will maintain the skin's healthy pH (the acidity level)

• Moisturizing cream, which should be hypo allergenic. This will prevent dangerous itching of dry and delicate skin. Avoid at all costs scratching that itch!

• Protective creams and ointments can protect skin from wetness and soothe the skin thereby speeding up the healing process and preventing possible rashes.

Maintaining good skin condition with these products will also help avoid small breaks in the skin that could lead to ulcer formation.

General skin care tips:

• Ensure adequate bathing or showering to keep skin clean.

• Be sure not to spend too long in the bath and do not use very hot water (this can deplete natural moisture from the skin).

• Towel dry gently to avoid damaging the skin.

• Avoid harsh cleaning agents that can irritate the skin.

• Try to avoid perspiration.

• Regularly inspect the skin for warning signs such as redness, burning sensations or pain. Consult the nurse or physician immediately if you suspect a problem.

4. PAIN MANAGEMENT

Physicians and nurses as well as front line health workers have to ask the right questions to pinpoint the extent of the pain problem. For example: "Can you describe the pain?" "What makes the pain better?" Try to initiate an honest, open conversation on pain issues.

Quality of life research studies have consistently highlighted that pain is an overwhelming issue for patients living with a leg ulcer. It is unfortunate that sometimes patients accept the pain as the norm, believing "it comes with the territory." Further research has also shown that health workers and even professionals assume that venous leg ulcers are not painful.

Venous leg ulcers are painful because nerve endings are exposed; a moist, occlusive dressing will protect the nerves and can reduce pain. Furthermore, the pain from engorged veins and swollen tissue in the legs can usually be reduced by compression from bandages or stockings and from elevating the legs.

To relieve local pain associated with chronic venous leg ulcers, the non narcotic varieties of pain killers such as ibuprofen or acetaminophen usually help.

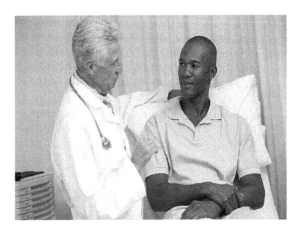

HEALING TIME

There are several factors that will influence how quickly you can expect a leg ulcer to heal.

In general the smaller the ulcer when treatment begins, the faster it will heal. This means it is important to seek medical help as soon as you suspect a problem.

Ulcers that are more than six months old will heal more slowly than those that are treated earlier.

The more serious the underlying venous problem the longer it will take for the ulcer to heal and the more aggressive treatment will be needed.

EIGHT SELF HELP TIPS

1. KEEP THE COMPRESSION BANDAGING IN PLACE

Instructions given by the nurse or physician as well as those provided by the manufacturer should be followed conscientiously regarding managing the compression bandage between visits.

The bandage should be applied like a sleeve not a clamp, otherwise it can create a tourniquet effect and this can cause pain. Avoid producing a high band of compression in the calf region of the leg which is a common mistake.

If the bandage has to be reapplied in the morning, make sure it is done before the person gets up or after he or she has been lying down for at least half an hour.

The more time the patient spends under good compression the more time the ulcer has to actively try to repair itself. Each time a little swelling is allowed to occur it must be reduced to start the healing process again. For this reason the medical team may decide on a system that stays on for a full week.

Check with the person in your care to see if there are some instructions she does not understand. Find out if she knows why compression is important. If she does not understand, explain the reasoning behind this treatment.

2. EXERCISE

Veins do not have their own muscles to pump blood out of the leg. For this reason they rely on us to use our foot and leg muscles to provide the pumping force.

Exercise without compression works against the treatment by forcing more blood into the lower leg and raising the venous pressure.

3. ELEVATE THE LEGS AND REST PROPERLY

Lie down and raise your feet higher than your heart by about six inches. This removes the problem of gravity trying to slow down the venous blood moving up your legs. Instead gravity is now working gently in your favor. Do this type of resting as frequently as possible.

4. USE COMPRESSION STOCKINGS CORRECTLY

After the leg ulcer has healed or before one develops the use of these stockings is vital to prevent swelling in the legs and therefore help prevent leg ulcers and venous problems.

Read the manufacturer's instructions and ensure proper fitting with a specialist fitter.

For best results, compression stockings should be worn from dawn till dusk, all day long, every day.

They should be put on in the morning before getting out of bed. If the patient has left his bed without putting the stockings on, he should go back, lie down for a few minutes with his legs elevated and wiggle his toes. He should remain in this position and then pull on the stockings.

Over a time, due to swelling or becoming more muscular, a person may need to change the type of compression stockings he or she is using. Keep a record of the size of the stocking, and make a note of the stockings purchased, pinpointing the date for purchasing new ones.

A commonly asked question is, "Should you remove stockings if aching or tightness in the leg is experienced?" The answer is usually, No. The reasons for the symptoms are due probably to a period of inactivity and a build-up of fluid in the leg. Walking around or exercising the legs is recommended.

Compression stockings should be washed by hand in cool water with a mild soap. Wring them gently in a towel and avoid stretching them. Let them dry in the open air, away from sources of heat. And NEVER put them in the dryer.

5. ADHERE TO TREATMENT

Whether the person in your care is having surgery, taking medication, having stockings fitted and so on, she must fully understand what she needs to do to help herself.

6. MAINTAIN ADEQUATE SKIN CARE

As well as following the tips and using the recommended products, the skin must be inspected on a regular basis. Any changes or suspected problems should be reported immediately to the medical team. Remember, small fresh ulcers can heal quickly so the sooner they are detected and treated the less discomfort, bother and expense will be involved.

7. ASK FOR PAIN TREATMENT

Pain is a major quality of life issue and there is no need for the sufferer to accept pain as normal.

8. CHOOSE A HEALTHY LIFESTYLE

If you smoke, stop; eat nutritiously, lose weight if necessary, seek support from family, friends and caregivers, and maintain a positive attitude.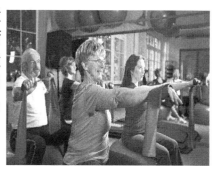

SEVEN COMMON SENSE TIPS

1. AVOID STANDING FOR LONG PERIODS OF TIME

If your job or certain activities demand you stand without moving for long periods of time, this will usually increase swelling and hinder the healing process. You must try to be assertive and ensure that you rest properly or obtain a chair or stool. Try to move about as often as possible and exercise the legs. Sitting in cramped quarters can also be a problem which should be avoided.

2. DO NO HARM

A knock on your ulcer can set back the healing process significantly. Even damage to skin that is vulnerable to leg ulcer development can bring on the condition.

Do not expose your legs to strong heat sources – this is a common mistake as people often think heat will help circulation. Instead, the heat can damage skin and veins.

Try to arrange your surroundings so that they are as accident free as possible. Get rid of protruding objects, make sure the floors are not slippery, and so on.

3. DON'T CROSS YOUR LEGS

When sitting or lying down do not cross your legs. It can reduce circulation and therefore worsen the venous problems.

4. AVOID WEARING RESTRICTIVE CLOTHING

Tight pants, tight socks, garters or anything that can restrict blood flow must be avoided.

5. MAINTAIN GOOD HYGIENE & INFECTION CONTROL

If you are involved with dressing changes or any activity around the leg ulcer make sure you have washed your hands thoroughly. An infection caused by unclean hands can seriously set you back as far as the healing process is concerned.

6. AVOID SCRATCHING

This is the most common way of bringing on a leg ulcer by your own actions. Often scratching can be due to dry itchy skin and there are products available that can rectify this. You may scratch without thinking so make sure your nails are kept short to minimize damage.

7. TRAVEL TIPS

When riding in the car, stop, get out and walk around frequently to avoid build-up of fluid in the legs.

If you sit for a long period of time in the same position on an airplane, try to get up and walk about or do the foot exercises. Informing the attendant of your needs may help you obtain a seat with more leg room or better access to the aisle.

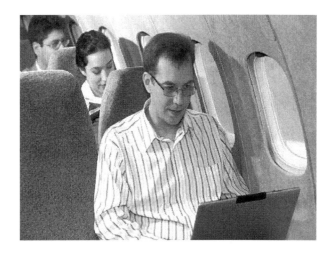

ASSESSMENT CHECKLIST

Tick any you need to action:

Self help tips

Compression	❏
Leg elevation	❏
Adherence to treatment	❏
Compression stockings	❏
Skin care	❏
Pain relief	❏

Lifestyle changes

Quitting smoking	❏
Nutrition	❏
Weight loss	❏
Family/caregiver	❏
support	❏
Positive attitude	❏

Common sense tips

Avoid standing	❏
Do no harm	❏
Avoid crossing legs	❏
Avoid restrictive clothing	❏
No scratching	❏
Good hygiene	❏
Travel tips	❏

CASE EXAMPLE

Seventy-six-year-old Mrs. M. owned a hair salon for many years. She is retired now and is visited frequently by family members but she has Parkinson's disease and sometimes has difficulty walking. For the past three months she has had a venous leg ulcer and complains of pain 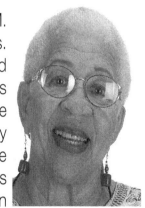 and aching around the ulcer. On your first visit with Mrs. M. you notice she's not wearing compression stockings or a compression bandage and recently she aggravated the ulcer with a fall.

What are the issues here?

What advice and help would you give Mrs. M.?

YOUR ANSWERS TO CASE EXAMPLE

SUGGESTED ANSWERS TO CASE EXAMPLE

What are the issues here?

Standing for long periods of time is a known risk factor for developing venous ulcers, and Mrs. M. would have done just that during her years as a hairdresser. That should encourage her not to stand for long periods now that she doesn't have to.

Because the ulcer seems well established and there may be a long healing time involved, it would seem necessary she should be educated, motivated and trained to help herself when it comes to adhering to treatment and knowing how to relieve her symptoms.

The fact that she has Parkinson's disease is another risk factor when it comes to damaging her ulcer while walking. It may also prevent her from getting enough exercise to help her blood circulation.

What advice and help would you give Mrs. M.?

You should address the pain and aching problem by checking she has appropriate pain medication and is taking it as prescribed. Secondly, explain that raising her legs 6 inches above her heart while lying down on the couch can bring relief of both pain and aching in the leg.

Check with the health professional to find out if she should be wearing a compression bandage or stocking; if so, always check and encourage her to wear the compression treatment.

Check out the surrounding furniture and reduce risk areas where her walking problems due to Parkinson's disease may cause her to accidentally damage her legs.

CONCLUSION

The root cause of venous leg ulcers is the swelling of the legs caused by high venous blood pressure. Prevent the swelling and you are controlling the disease. This means that for people with venous ulcers, the most important aspect of treatment and prevention is effective compression of the legs through bandaging or stockings.

Although all the self help tips and adherence to treatment are vital for healing and prevention, the morale and well being of the patient is also very important.

Caregivers, family members and medical staff should listen, nurture and communicate effectively and always ensure any pain issue is addressed.

Patients should be encouraged to take some ownership of the treatment by way of being assertive, asking questions and making sure there they thoroughly understand the issues. There are many players in the medical team and the only way to ensure success is for you to participate in all the preventative and treatment actions necessary for good health.

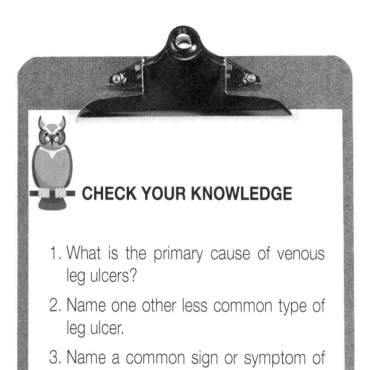

CHECK YOUR KNOWLEDGE

1. What is the primary cause of venous leg ulcers?

2. Name one other less common type of leg ulcer.

3. Name a common sign or symptom of venous leg ulcers.

4. What is the most effective treatment and prevention of a venous leg ulcer?

5. Name one self-help tip for a person suffering from a venous leg ulcer.

TEST YOURSELF

Please circle to indicate the best answer:

1. Why is the word "venous" used to describe this type of leg ulcer?

a. The underlying problem causing a leg ulcer is due to vein problems.

b. There is reduced oxygen to the leg tissues.

c. Venous denotes harmful swelling in the legs.

d. Indicates there is reddish skin staining around the ankle.

2. What is the most important treatment for venous ulcers?

a. The correct wound dressing choice

b. The Ankle Brachial Pressure Index (ABPI)

c. Compression therapy

d. Antibiotics

3. Which of the following is NOT a sign of a venous ulcer?

a. Swelling around the leg

b. Pain relieved when leg is elevated

c. Reddish-brown staining on leg and ankles

d. Loss of sensation or feeling in the foot

4. Which of the following is NOT a form of compression therapy?

a. Pumps

b. Stockings/hosiery

c. Bandages

d. Hydrogel dressings

5. What can cause swelling in the legs and ankles?

a. Tight stockings

b. Gravity causing more blood in the lower leg

c. High pressure in the veins causing fluid to leak

d. Too high a room temperature

6. Which of the following should you NOT do with a patient?

a. Ask about any pain caused by the venous ulcer.

b. Help direct the right amount of heat from a lamp to the ulcer.

c. Help avoid scratching the skin by using moisturizers.

d. Encourage elevating the leg when appropriate.

7. Which of the following statements is NOT true for using of compression stockings?

a. Stockings work collaboratively with the calf muscles for a dual effect.

b. There are different compression levels for different stockings.

c. Only compression bandages reduce actual pain and swelling.

d. Stockings prevent further fluid build-up in the leg.

ANSWERS

1. a. The underlying problems causing a leg ulcer are due to vein problems. Reduced oxygen, harmful swelling and staining of the skin are all factors related to venous leg ulcers but are not related to the term "venous."

2. c. Compression therapy is the "gold standard" treatment through bandaging, stocking or a compression pump.

3. d. Loss of sensation or feeling in the foot is actually a major symptom of diabetic foot ulcers.

4. d. Neither Hydrogel dressings nor any other type of dressing provides any therapeutic compression pressure around the leg.

5. d. High pressure in the veins causing fluid to leak can cause swelling in the legs and ankles. Gravity does contribute to the problem but is not the direct technical cause of the swelling.

6. b. It is not recommended for any heat to be applied to an ulcer by way of fire, sun, Jacuzzi, saunas, etc.

7. c. Although stockings are not as aggressive as compression treatment, they do still reduce actual pain and swelling.

REFERENCES

Brooks, J, Ersser, SJ, Lloyd, A., & Ryan, TJ (2004). Nurse-led education sets out to improve patient concordance and prevent recurrence of leg ulcers. Journal of Wound Care, 13(3), 111-116.

Charles, H. (2002). Venous leg ulcer pain and its characteristics. Journal of Tissue Viability, 12(4), 154-158.

Davies, B. & Edwards, N. (2004). RNs measure effectiveness of best practice guidelines. Registered Nurse Journal, 16 (1), 21-23.

McGuckin, M., Williams, L., Brooks, J., & Cherry, G. (2001). Guidelines in practice: the effect on healing of venous ulcers. Advances in Skin & Wound Care, 14, 33-36.

Nelson, EA, Iglesias, CP, Cullum, N., & Torgerson, DJ (2004). Randomized clinical trial of four-layer and short-stretch compression bandages for venous leg ulcers (VenUS I). British Journal of Surgery, 91, 1292-1299.

Nemeth, KA, Harrison, MB, Graham, ID, & Burke, S. (2004). Understanding venous leg ulcer pain: results of a longitudinal study. Ostomy/Wound Management, 50(1), 34-46.

Padberg, FT, Johnston, MV, & Sisto, SA (2004). Structured exercise improves calf muscle pump function in chronic venous insufficiency: a randomized trial. Journal of Vascular Surgery, 39, 79-87.

Palfreyman, SJ, Nelson, EA, Lochiel, R., & Michaels, JA (2007). Dressings for healing venous leg ulcers. The Cochrane Database of Systematic Reviews, Issue 1. John Wiley & Sons, Ltd.

Polignano, R., Bonadeo, P., Gasbarro, S., & Allegra, C. (2004). A randomised controlled study of four-layer compression versus Unna's Boot for venous ulcers. Journal of Wound Care, 13(1), 21-24.

Registered Nurses' Association of Ontario (2007). Assessment and Management of Pain (Revised). Toronto, Ontario: Registered Nurses' Association of Ontario.

Sibbald, RG, Orsted, HL, Coutts, PM, & Keast, DH (2006). Best practice recommendations for preparing the wound bed: Update 2006. Wound Care Canada, 4, 15-29.

Printed in Great Britain
by Amazon